The more
healthy
and
better
YOU

Table Of Contents

Chapter 1: Introduction about Healthy Lifestyle

A healthier, happier and more successful you

You can become a healthier, happier and more successful person by making a few simple changes to your lifestyle. You will have to make changes to the overall you, not just change the amount of exercise you do or your diet. The secret to achieving happiness and a healthier you is to balance your body and mind in harmony, it is only when we are balanced in physical health, mental and spiritual that we are truly healthy.

If we are healthy then we are happier and can reach success more easily in life, here are some ways you can bring back harmony and balance to your life

Exercise is an essential part, it helps to tone our body, keep our heart and lungs healthy and detoxifies. Exercise can be anything from more vigorous routines such as aerobics to simply walking, pick your favorite activity and set aside a specific time of day and commit yourself to devoting a half-hour per day towards getting your body back into shape.

Eating right is the next essential step to maintaining a well-balanced life; our bodies need the right amount of vitamins, nutrients and minerals to work at its best. Making changes to our diet is easy, keep away from fast foods which contain a lot of saturated fats and sugar and start including more whole grains, chicken, fish, plenty of green vegetables and try to eat fresh fruit instead of juice when available.

Along with making changes to your diet you should include supplements such as vitamins, nutrients and minerals. Modern farming methods strip many of our foods of the minerals our bodies require and now just provide us with the basic nutrients. Due to this we might be lacking in certain minerals and vitamins, by supplementing your diet with vitamin and mineral supplements we can ensure we still get all the vital minerals, nutrients and vitamins we need in our daily diet.

Reducing the amount of stress we have in our life plays an important part in how we are able to cope with it. Stress can do much damage to our body and mind and has been linked with "burnout", fatigue, sleep problems, depression and it lowers our immune system. Learning techniques on how to cope with stress and worry are essential to keeping yourself balanced and full of energy. There are a wide variety of techniques from simple breathing exercises which can be done anywhere, at anytime, to yoga which is a full system for relaxation and de-stressing to meditation. There are many books, DVDS and CDS available on the subject or there are courses you can attend.

Lastly but by no means the least important is keeping life fun, doing something which you enjoy doing and makes you feel relaxed and happy each day. No you are not being selfish by taking time out each day just for yourself, this time is essential. It is just as important as exercising, eating right and reducing stress, your time could be spent doing a hobby or pastime that you enjoy, sitting quietly and reading, taking a hot bubble bath while listening to your favorite music or spending quality time with your family or friends. It can be anything as long as it's something you like to do and enjoying doing.

12 Tips for better health

The biggest step to aiming towards better health is admitting the fact that you need to make changes towards becoming healthier and fitter. Here are some tips to help you improve your health and help you to reach a new and improved you.

1. Make it a life goal to obtain a healthier outlook on life which will undoubtedly lead to a healthier you, if you are determined to reach a better state of health, making it a reality will be so much easier.

2. Support your new way of thinking by learning everything you can about ways of reaching better health and living a healthier lifestyle. You can use the internet, books, DVDS, clubs, gyms and support groups to your benefit, knowing all you can about healthy living gives you a great base to work from.

3. You have to start somewhere so start by taking a look at your kitchen and reorganizing in preparation for your new way of life. Reorganize your kitchen cabinets, cupboards and refrigerator to ensure that there are no signs of the old you and all the signs of the things that will help you in your new lifestyle.

4. Replace old food with your new healthier choice and don't forget to purchase any small appliances which you will need to support your healthier way of eating, such as blenders and food weighing scales.

5. Get a large planner calendar, pin it up in your kitchen and mark the day when you choose to begin your new lifestyle and stick to it no matter what.

6. From day one keep a journal, this can either be a traditional one or use your computer. You should include all thoughts and feelings about your new ways along with all the changes you see about yourself. This is essential to look back on to see the positive changes that are occurring due to your positive outlook and changes you have made.

7. Positive thoughts and self talk or affirmations are a necessity; they will give you confidence at the beginning and will continue to take you through the tough times which will often occur during the early changes.

8. Along with changes to your diet you will also have to make changes to the amount of exercise you do per day, while good healthy food is essential, exercise is also just as important to help ward off the onset of diseases such as heart disease, as well as helping us to firm up our body or lose a few pounds.

9.   Give up any bad habits such as smoking or drinking, you will never reach your optimal peak of health while you are puffing away on cigarettes or drinking on a regular basis.

10.   Make sure that you get the recommended 5 portions of fruit and veggies per day on your new regime, fruit and veggies are packed full of essential vitamins.

11.   Make sure you learn ways to eliminate as much stress from your lifestyle as you possibly can, there are many ways to do this with one of them sure to be suitable for your situation.

12.   Cut out excess salt, sugar and fatty foods from your diet, this will effectively lower your cholesterol and blood pressure.

Notes on Nutrition

The best place to begin taking notes about nutrition is with the United States Department of Agriculture (USDA). The USDA offers recommendations about what they find to be healthy eating-related habits for the general public. And their information covers these main areas of focus: nutrition pyramid, needed nutrients, weight management, physical fitness and food safety.

Nutrition Pyramid

The USDA has revised dietary guidelines and lists a food pyramid with color scheme to help people eat in a healthy manner.

Needed Nutrients

The USDA advises people to drink and eat a wide variety of nutrient-dense beverages and foods from the basic food groups they note in their nutrition pyramid. They also suggest limiting alcohol, salt, added sugars, cholesterol, saturated and trans fats. And they recommend following plans like the Dietary Approaches to Stop Hypertension (DASH) Eating Plan or their USDA Food Guide.

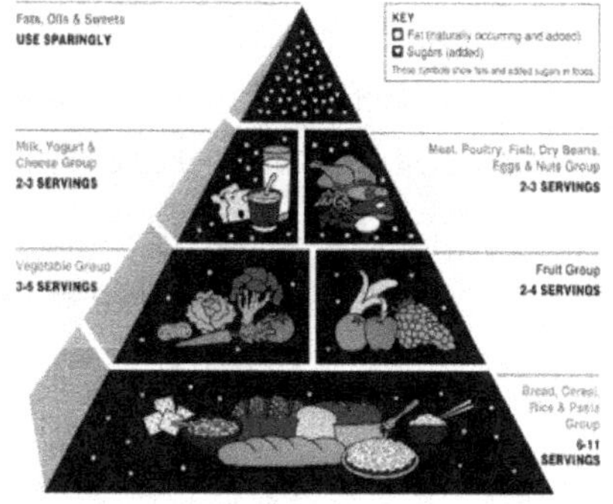

Weight Management

The general weight focus of the USDA stresses that people strive to maintain body weight in a healthy range, balancing calories from beverages and foods with those expended. And to help manage weight control as aging occurs, people are to gradually decrease the amounts of foods and beverages consumed and increase physical fitness.

Physical Fitness

The USDA desires people to regularly partake in physical activity while decreasing sedentary activities in order to promote not only healthy bodies but overall general health and psychological well-being. Optimum activity is targeted at around 30 -90 minutes minimum a day of moderate to intense physical, depending upon weight status, age and eating habits. For even more health benefits, a combination of either more intense activity and / or longer periods of activity is advised for most persons instead of just 30 minutes, checking with healthcare providers first for approval.

Key areas of focus for physical fitness are stretching exercises for increased flexibility, cardiovascular conditioning and calisthenics or resistance exercises to improve endurance and muscles.

Food Safety

The USDA recommends that people avoid microbial food borne illnesses by thoroughly washing hands, surfaces where food is handled and vegetables and fruits. They also advise against washing meats and poultry; however, separate raw foods from those that are already cooked or ready to eat when shopping, handling and storing foods.

They also recommend that foods need to be cooked at temperatures safe enough to destroy microorganisms and promptly stored in refrigeration or freezers if perishable.
And they advise people to avoid:

- Raw or unpasteurized milk
- Products created from unpasteurized milk
- raw or partially cooked eggs
- Foods containing raw eggs
- Raw or undercooked poultry and meats
- Unpasteurized juices
- Raw sprouts.

Chapter II: Look Good, Feel Better

How we look on the outside very often reflects how we feel on the inside, if we know we look good on the outside and are getting praise and compliments this automatically gives us a boost and makes us feel good on the inside. Ways to looking better on the outside and ultimately feeling better on the inside include dieting, eating a well balanced diet, exercising, and taking general care of your body and also taking care of your mental health.

Staying active

Keeping active by exercising not only helps you to lose those few extra pounds but also tones your muscles leaving you looking better but also feeling healthier by helping to ward off diseases. There are many forms of exercise and it doesn't have to be expensive, you can buy cheap basic gym equipment to use in your own home or even take up a form of great exercise which doesn't cost a penny, walking. In order to maintain the peak of health you should aim to exercise for at least 30 minutes per day every day of the week while maintaining a healthy balanced diet.

Eating right

A well balanced diet consists of eating at the right times without snacking in-between and eating plenty of fresh fruit and veg, which are rich in vitamins and minerals. If you are trying to lose a few pounds then it is essential that you don't eat more calories per day than you are burning off and cutting down on foods rich in salt, fats and carbohydrates is essential to maintaining a healthy body. A well balanced diet is considered to be one that includes bread, cereals, fish, lean meat, chicken, potatoes, and dairy products, this along with exercise not only makes you look better but can help to counteract the onset of many health related problems.

Taking general care of your body includes numerous small things which go towards making you look good, for example having a make over by way of changing your old hairstyle, getting it cut and dyed can make a huge difference to how you feel and give you a much needed boost. Paying a visit to a manicurist or pedicurist will give your hands and nails a treat, having your teeth whitened at the dentist can give you good reason to smile more. It's all the little things that can come together to make a big difference that you have to take into account when looking for ways to make you feel better on the outside.

Mental health is important too

Your mental health, your feelings and thoughts can also make a huge difference to how you feel on the outside and inside. If you have negative thoughts and feelings on the whole then your outlook will be one of negativity that leads to low self-confidence and low self-image. Daily affirmations can help you to change your pattern of thinking and help you gain self-confidence and are an enormous confidence booster.

All of the above when combined together can lead to a healthier and happier person who not only looks good on the outside and oozes self-confidence, but is also healthier and fitter on the inside with a better outlook on life in general and so is better able to cope with life.

The Importance of Maintaining a Healthy Weight

Being overweight not only looks unsightly and makes you feel less attractive it also poses a far greater risk, a risk to your health. Therefore, there are many reasons why it is important that you maintain a healthy weight by eating well-balanced meals and getting regular exercise. Being over weight has been linked with many conditions affecting not only our physical health but also our mental health, studies have shown that those people who are overweight and don't get regular exercise are more at risk of developing depression than those that exercise on a regular basis and eat a well balanced and varied diet. Experts have agreed that the more overweight a person is then the more likely they are to suffer severe health problems, however once the person takes steps to start losing weight and changes their lifestyle, then the percentage starts to drop. If you are overweight then even just by losing 10 or 20 pounds you can begin to reduce the increased associated risks to your health and make improvements. You should defiantly consider losing weight if you are overweight and any of the following conditions apply to you.

If there is a history in your family of certain chronic diseases – people who have relatives with heart conditions or diabetes have been known to develop these conditions if they are overweight.

There are any pre-existing medical conditions – high blood pressure, high cholesterol and levels of high sugar are all signs of illness due to being overweight.

Having an apple shape – if you carry more weight around your stomach then you are at a higher risk of developing diabetes, some forms of cancer or developing heart problems.'

Illness associated with being overweight

Problems with the gallbladder and especially gallstones

High blood pressure

Developing certain types of cancer

Developing diabetes

Developing gout

Developing problems with the breathing such as sleep apnea, which causes a person to pause when breathing while asleep

Chest problems such as asthma or bronchitis

Gallbladder problems

Although it is not clear why, being overweight can have an affect on the gallbladder, gallstones are a very common problem in someone who is overweight and causes severe problems with those who are obese.

Heart disease

If you are overweight you are twice as likely to suffer from high blood pressure that is the major cause of and a big risk factor in heart disease and strokes. Being overweight can lead to a condition known as angina, angina is felt as pain in the chest caused by a decrease in oxygen to the heart. If you are severely overweight or obese then this has been linked to causing sudden death without any warning signs from a stroke.

Diabetes

Being overweight has been linked to type 2 diabetes and is a known contributor to health death, heart disease and blindness; people who are overweight are twice as likely to suffer from type 2 diabetes as those people who are of normal weight.

Lowering your cholesterol

Keeping an eye on your cholesterol levels and maintaining a healthy level is essential if you want to remain healthy. There are many ways in which we can reduce the amount of cholesterol to ensure it remains at levels within the guidelines and to avoid illnesses such as heart disease. Here are some ways you can successfully lower your cholesterol level.

Changing your diet and eating your way to a lower cholesterol level is the easiest way, tips for doing this include:

Burn off at least as many calories as you eat during the course of a day

Make sure that you get at least 30 minutes of exercise every day of the week

Eat a wide variety of foods that are rich in nutrients

Include at least 5 portions of fruit and vegetables per day in your diet

Eat lost of high-fiber, wholegrain foods in your diet

Include fish in your diet at least twice a week

Cut foods poor in nutrients out of your diet

Cut down on the amount of trans-fat and saturated fat foods in your diet

Remove the skin from chicken and eat only lean meat in your diet

Only include fat free and low fat dairy products in your diet

In order to reduce trans fat in your diet cut out foods containing partially hydrogenated vegetable oil

Include very little or no salt in your diet

Only drink alcohol in moderation

- Always read nutritional labels on food

You can keep your levels of cholesterol under control by exercising on a regular basis and here are some tips for getting started on a fitness program:

Start off slowly and gradually build up until you are getting 30 minutes of exercise per day

Make your daily workout become a part of your life by doing it at the same time everyday whenever possible

Make sure you drink enough water to ensure that you don't dehydrate

Enjoy your workout by joining a gym or working out with a friend

Keep a journal of your workout and write down the benefits you feel after exercising

Walk instead of taking the elevator, leave the car at home or walk or cycle to work

Vary your routine, go swimming one day, cycling the next, walking e.t.c

If you feel unwell then take a break from exercising and pick up your routine when you are feeling better

You should also aim to make changes to your lifestyle in order to keep your levels of cholesterol down and here are some tips for making those changes:

Get nutritional and physical advice from a healthcare professional

Always read food labels so you know how much fat, sodium and other ingredients you are eating in your diet

If you smoke or drink then seriously consider giving up   .

Why Weight Watchers Doesn't Work

We have all heard of Weight Watchers and many of us who have struggled with diets with the need to lose a few pounds may have even tried attending Weight Watchers meetings, some have success while many others fail miserably. Weight watchers cannot work magic, just like any other form of dieting the success behind it is all down to the person not the plan to lose weight; sadly, there is no magic formula which will help us to shed the pounds overnight while we sleep. Understanding why any diet does not work is critical for success and the Weight Watchers program is no exception, so why do so many of us fail when it comes to dieting and following a program such as Weight Watchers?

Persevering with the plan
The biggest mistake that many of us make is not sticking to the plan, a program such as Weight Watchers requires you to pay a membership fee so it

is essential that you have the commitment needed to go into the plan and follow it through by sticking to it before signing up for membership. Weight Watchers relies on the person keeping track of what they eat and taking full advantage of the support that Weight Watchers gives to members. All diets basically rely on counting calories or points, values of the food we eat and weight watchers relies on a points system, a point value is assigned to each food based on the amount of calories and fat content within that particular food. A person is then allowed a certain number of points throughout the day based on their sex and weight, the system of course will work adequately if the number of points are stuck to per day but if the person continually goes over the recommended daily allotted amount of points then quite simply they are not going to lose weight and indeed could in fact gain weight.

Failing to keep a journal
It is essential for a plan such as Weight Watchers to be successful that you keep a journal and write down all the foods and keep a count of all the points which you are eating throughout the day, simply relying on your memory to keep count is not good enough. Besides simply forgetting you ate something you could also conveniently forget all about that nibble you had with your coffee, if you are going to be successful with the Weight Watchers program then you have to keep a written journal and include every single point that you put through your lips.

Guesswork
One of the biggest reasons why so many people fail at Weight Watchers is they underestimate the number of points they have eaten throughout a day. By guessing the number of points in a plateful of food you are on the track to failure, by repeatedly underestimating the number of points you are eating and by doing this you can never expect to lose weight. Some people who follow the weight watchers system also misunderstand the system because certain foods such as vegetables have no points as long as you measure that amount in one cup. However they get misled into thinking that you are allowed as many vegetables as you wish and its still classed as no points, therefore some people think they are allowed to eat an unlimited amount of these types of food which is wrong. Always be sure you totally understand the points system of a program like Weight Watchers and if in doubt ask a representative for advice on calculating using the points system.

Any type of diet requires willpower and determination and Weight Watchers is no exception, only by following the guidelines set out will you be successful in your weight loss program, proper calculation of points and keeping a written account if everything you eat is essential to making the program work as is sticking with it over time and changing your lifestyle and the way you eat after you have successfully lost the amount of weight you want to lose.

Drop and Give Me 10! Ways to Lose 10 Lbs.

Sometimes you just want to kick start an exercise program into gear or lose some weight in order to look good for an upcoming family or other event or just to feel better and fit into your clothes better. For those and any other occasions, it sure would be nice to lose 10 lbs fast. Well, help is here with tips form the pros who've been there, done that. So dig in and drop 10!

Make Time
Make no more excuses! Your health and fitness is priority and there is no better time than now to lose. If you do not set aside time and schedule fitness goals into your regular daily plans, you are not planning to succeed, but rather failing to plan. So grab your day planner and calendar, and jot down at least 30 minutes a day for working out with physical fitness activities.

Plan Your 'Fat' Attack
Next do a little homework and plan your attack on those extra fat pounds. You can choose among many popular fitness and weight loss plans like Weight Watchers, the Suzanne Somers Weight Loss Program, the Mayo Clinic Plan, Atkins, Bill Philips Body for Life Program, Jenny Craig, Slim-Fast and more. Or you can head to your local gym and hire a trainer or just get moving on your own, noting reps, and resistance for increased endurance and strength training.

Mental Mindset
Make an attitude adjustment so that you have a positive, healthy outlook for your fitness goals. For help getting this mindset and keeping it going throughout your program, head to your local library for motivational and inspirational books, audio cassettes, DVDs, videos and articles. Also look on the Internet for helpful tools: articles, ezines, MP3 and other audio files, video clips, ebooks, reports and training.

Change Your Diet
Take charge of your nutritional needs by setting up a good diet or choosing a good diet plan. A good place to look online is at eDiets.com where many popular diet plans are linked up for you offering recipes, a community forum for reaching out to new healthy friends online, meal planning and journaling and a lot more. Head to the library for helpful materials, too, and other dietary and nutritional sites online.

Track Your Journey to Success
Grab a notebook and journey your way to your goals and beyond. Clearly write out what you want to accomplish, by what date and how you intend to get there using what methods, for instance: working out 30 minutes a day and eating right following the Weight Watchers program guidelines.

Fitness with Friends
Make friends and help support each other along the way. Search "fitness forum" on the Internet to locate free places to register and chat away.

Set Realistic Goals
Get real and focus on what works best like losing 2 lbs per week. Losing more any faster often results in the pounds returning.

Using Your Weight Loss Plan to Help Others

If you have been successful at devising and sticking to a weight loss plan then you should share your plan and success with others who are striving to have the same success as you. There is nothing like motivation to encourage others to stick to it and succeed and if they see it working then they are more likely to be want to stick with a plan too and gain the same success in their life. Sharing and motivating each other is the number one reason why weight loss clubs such as weight watchers have such a high success rate, knowing you are not the only one out there who is struggling and needs to shed a pounds can make a huge difference just by giving the confidence a boost. So if you have been successful in your weight loss plan then what can you do to get it out there and share it with others, here are ideas to get you started.

Write a blog
The Internet is an excellent place to write a blog and it enables you to get your thoughts and ideas out there to millions of people throughout the world, there are many websites that now offer free blog space and this is ideal for getting your information out. A blog space can be thought of like an online diary, your space to share thoughts, feelings and ideas and you spread it by word of mouth all over the world. Use your blog space to share your successful weight loss plan and write down all that it took to get you where you are today in detail. You can include the plan you used along with exercise routines and menus that you followed along as well as your thoughts and feelings as you went through the plan to encourage people that dieting can work.

Have weekly meetings
If you know a group of friends who are wanting to diet then get together and hire a local meeting hall weekly or alternate going to different homes every week for a diet club meeting. Getting together once a week means you can all get weighed together at the same time, share your highlights and console those who have faltered throughout the week. Keep written records for all members of the group and plot your progress weekly, if one of you has been particularly successful in the past with your weight loss plan then maybe you are the one to lead the group and encourage other members to follow the same plan you did.

Write an e-book
If you have had great success on your weight loss plan then consider writing a small e-book about your experiences and success in order to encourage others. It doesn't have to be anything fancy and all computers come with word processing software, start by mapping out from the introduction, then go through various chapters and when you have finished print it out and distribute it among friends, it's a great, fun way to get your success story out there and to give others the encouragement they might need.

Chapter III: Be Active to Maintain Health

Walking Your Way to a Healthier You

Walking is the best form of exercise you can have to obtain better health and a fitter you and it will cost you nothing. It is a form of exercise which can be taken up by anyone regardless of age or physical condition providing you start off sensibly, as with all forms of exercise you are not used to doing.

The first steps to getting healthier should be taken slowly and it is advisable if you do not exercise on a regular basis to start off with no more than a 10-minute walk most days of the week. This can then be gradually increased to walking 3 times a day for 10 minutes or twice a day for 15 minutes at a time. There are many ways you can fit this into your daily routine without too much trouble; just consider when and where you could alter your routine to walk instead of taking the car or bus.

The benefits of walking are numerous to your health and wellbeing and simply by altering your routine and walking 30 minutes or more each and every day you can

- See an increase in your overall fitness and the tone of your muscles
- Feel good and look better
- Find that your level of energy increases
- Feel a lot less stressed and are slower to start feeling stressed
- Find that your pattern of sleep changes and you sleep better and feel more rested on waking
- Begin to reduce the risk of heart disease
- Reduce the risk of developing certain types of cancer
- Find that depression starts lifting and you don't feel down as easily as you once did
- Your outlook on life in general and the way you deal with things changes for the better
- You lose weight and look better
- You find that your muscles, joints and bones are stronger
- You reduce the risk of developing diabetes

You can start gaining all these and more benefits simply by increasing the amount of walking you do per day and being more active. In order to gain the best health and fitness from walking you should aim to walk at a moderate pace, a moderate pace means that while you shouldn't be over exerting yourself you should be walking faster than strolling along. This means that while you are walking, you should be able to hold a conversation without getting breathless and your temperature should rise a little, but you shouldn't be sweating to the extreme.

Not only will you feel better and look better once you have been on your new regime for a while, you will feel many more benefits health wise and be well on the way to leading a more productive, happier and healthier way of lifestyle.

Running for Success

Running isn't just for runners anymore. Running just three days a week for 30 minutes has been proven to help maintain healthy weight as well as improve attitude and motivation. In short, running can help you become happier, healthier and more successful to. Here's how.

For Health
Running is not just an athlete's sport. Although you probably won't win the Boston Marathon, running can be a very healthy activity whether you choose to compete in races or not. In order to achieve optimal health benefits from running, you will want to work yourself up to a level of being able to run at least 30 minutes at a stretch, three or four days a week.

The best part about running is that you can do it anywhere with just a pair of good shoes. Go to your local running store and have them fit you into the right pair to ensure that you don't cause injury from inadequate shoes. The key here is not to have the cheapest shoes, the most expensive shoes or the nicest looking shoes, but to have the right shoes for your feet.

For Attitude
Running, above many other sports, can help develop a happier, healthier attitude towards life. If you can motivate yourself to get out there to run three days a week, you can do anything. Most people find that after they have been running for a few weeks that it becomes addicting. You will enjoy the control you have over yourself and will crave more. It can be most rewarding when you get out on the streets in inclement weather and brave a drizzle or windy day. The lessons you learn from running will help you be a more positive person and will teach you that anything is possible if you put your mind to it.

If you run with a negative attitude, you'll find that you won't get very far or you will walk a great chunk of the way. In order to convince yourself to keep on running, you'll find yourself telling yourself positive things, looking forward to the hills and forcing yourself to think that running is your favorite activity, even if it isn't. The amazing thing that will start to happen is that you will start to believe it. After awhile, you won't be forcing yourself to run, you really will enjoy it and look forward to it.

Once you reach this level, you will find yourself with a more positive attitude towards just about everything. Running is one of the best attitude adjustments there is. Once you start to look forward to running up those hills because it is going to make you stronger and faster, you'll find yourself thinking positively about all aspects of your life such as dealing with problem clients at work. Instead of getting irritated, you will begin to think about what you could say to calm them down, make them happy and move on to the next client.

For Motivation
After you conquer the first 30 minutes of non-stop running, you will probably
find yourself wondering if you could run further or faster. Most people can find
a 5k or 10k race within driving distance almost every weekend and this can
help you gauge how fast you can run. These races can serve as a great
motivator for you and your newfound hobby. Run your first one without regard
for time, just finish. After that, you will probably find yourself looking to
improve your personal best and you will easily be able to find more races
whenever you are ready to challenge yourself.

Cycling to your way to fitness

To gain benefits from cycling you don't have to be super fit, an athlete or
anything of the sort. The benefits of bicycling are great and it is a fun way to
get that much needed exercise.

Weight loss and bicycling
If you are trying to shed a few pounds, dieting alone very rarely works out in
the long term, however doing more exercise on a regular basis works
wonders. If you cycle on a daily basis then it will not only help you burn a
large number of calories during your workout but it will also raise your
metabolism and help you burn more calories throughout the day. Cycling
along a flat road or path at 12 mph will help you to burn off roughly 450
calories an hour, and even when you stop your metabolism is still speeding
ahead, helping to you burn calories quicker.

Not only can cycling help you to lose weight and keep it off, it is also beneficial
health wise. By cycling at least 20 miles per week you can help to reduce the
risk of developing heart disease by half compared to those who don't cycle.

Health benefits of bicycling
Cycling is classed as an aerobic form of exercise; this is a type of exercise
that is particularly beneficial to the lungs and heart. Your lungs expand with
the effort of pedaling, which allows you to get more oxygen into your body;
this in turn makes your heart beat faster to send the oxygen throughout your
body. If you develop powerful lungs and a strong heart then you are well and
truly on your way to fitness.

Just by cycling a few miles per day you will soon begin to feel fitter and
healthier, you will see your muscles beginning to tone. You thigh, backside
and calf muscles will gain the biggest benefit from cycling, as these are the
muscles that you will use the most, but overall you will find yourself in much
better shape. Perhaps you will find that you no longer get winded walking up
a flight of stairs. However, the best part is, that the more you bicycle, the
more you will enjoy it and look forward to your next outing.

Bicycling can also be beneficial when we are feeling down or if we suffer from
stress, anxiety or depression. When we exercise we release what are known
as endorphins into our bloodstream, endorphins bring about a feeling of
happiness and contentment and are a great way to combat stress and

depression. Cycling can be done almost anywhere by anyone, if you live in towns or the countryside there is always somewhere to bicycle. It doesn't have to be expensive and is a relatively safe sport, when you follow the few simple guidelines and can be enjoyed as a family.

Here are a few simple tips to help you get the most out of cycling

Always carry a puncture repair kit

Make sure you take a water bottle with you especially on long rides in the countryside

Keep your tires pumped up to the required level to make cycling easier

For safety always make sure you wear a bicycle helmet

Always have lights and reflectors on your bike to make sure you are seen

When cycling at night wear bright colors or preferably some sort of reflective material

Pilates for back pain

The most essential thing that those who suffer from back pain can learn is awareness of the neutral alignment of the spine and the strengthening of the postural muscles to support the alignment. For those people with back pain caused by the degeneration of discs and joints, or poor posture, a Pilate's exercise program can be beneficial to easing the problem.

Most back problems are caused by bad posture; this can be sitting, walking or standing. This causes us to lose strength in our postural muscles over time and gets worse until eventually you cannot even correct your posture if you want to. Pilates is an exellent form of exercise to remedy this problem too.

What is Pilates?
The Pilates method is a form of exercise that focuses on using the core postural muscles to help keep the body balanced and support the spine. It is a method that teaches awareness of breathing and alignment of the spine. In helping to prevent and alleviate back pain the system also strengthens the deep torso muscles.

While Pilates is a simple form of exercise you shouldn't underestimate the impact that it can have, Pilates can help to develop support for the deep postural muscles of the trunk. It brings an awareness of the importance of neutral alignment and leads to the shoulders and hips being suppler.

Pilates has roots in ballet and dance and as such some of the movements used in the system can be particularly challenging and difficult, however there are some exercises that can be learned and practiced at home between guided sessions. As when beginning any new form of exercise it is important that you seek the advice of your doctor before commencing, the instructor guiding the Pilates session should also be qualified.

One-on-one sessions may be the answer
For those who have significant back problems it may be advisable to have a few one-on-one sessions with an instructor qualified in Pilates and especially in treating those with back pain. While this is more expensive than attending a class it can be worth the extra expense to learn the exercise correctly by having one-on-one guidance.

While the exercises in the Pilates system should challenge you mentally and physically, they shouldn't cause you to struggle with them. If an exercise is causing you pain then it could be that you are not performing it correctly or it could be too difficult a position for you. You should make sure that you never put too much excessive stress on the intervertebral discs and avoid mental or physical fatigue.

As a general rule those suffering from back pain and attending Pilates should never perform any exercise that pushes the spine into extremes of extension or flexion. Side bending movements and twisting of the spine should also be avoided. As with most forms of exercise, it will take perseverance and some time spent attending classes before you will see any major improvements.

Chapter IV: Knowing Different Illness to Fight Them

Dealing with Chronic Illness

There are many challenges you will have to face when dealing with chronic illness. If you have been diagnosed with having a long lasting health condition, then understanding it and learning what you can do yourself to manage it, can help greatly.

Having a chronic illness doesn't have to mean that it is dangerous or deadly, asthma, diabetes and arthritis are all classed as chronic conditions that can be kept under control with medication and supervision. Providing you take care and have the proper treatment, people with these conditions can lead a normal life and are healthy for the majority of time. Although the underlying condition won't go away and is always there, it can be controlled successfully.

Many people who have conditions such as asthma don't consider themselves as having a chronic condition as they feel relatively well most of the time and think of their illness as more of a condition. However, a few people are affected not only physically but also emotionally, socially and for some even financially. The severity of the way it affects you is based on the severity of your condition and the treatment involved in your particular condition. However you are affected by your condition it will take time to accept and adjust to your chronic illness.

There is a certain process that everyone will go through whatever their illness, this is known as the coping process. When first diagnosed with chronic illness the person may have many different feelings, anger, worry, confusion and vulnerability are some of the most common feelings. The next stage to the coping process is the want to know and learn everything they can about their illness, by gaining insight and knowledge into their condition it makes it less frightening and they feel more in control.

The third stage is developing confidence in the treatment they have been given for their condition. Realizing that their medication or treatment will help to relieve symptoms and attacks such as those associated with asthma and low blood sugar levels. Over time managing the condition becomes second nature and worry and fear drop off as the person becomes more confident with their self-management.

Everyone will go through the stages of coping at their own rate, recognizing the various feelings and thoughts as you go through different stages is important and are all part of the coping process. To help you get through the coping process you should remember these tips.

Accept any feelings and thoughts – there are many emotions you may go through during the coping stage, it is important that you just let them come and go without giving them too much thought. Letting the feelings out by talking with someone can be a great release.

Ask questions and play an active role in self-care – make sure that you know everything about your illness that you possibly can, the unknown can be frightening, but what we know we can deal with much better. Learn what you can do to help your condition and what to do during the bad times of it.

Talk about your condition – remember other family members or loved ones will probably be going through similar feelings as you are after the diagnosis. Talk with family members and loved ones about your condition, don't leave them out of the loop

Keep a perspective – when first diagnosed it can be easy to let your illness take over your life and become the most important thing, keep things in perspective and carry on living your life just as you did before.

Understanding and preventing asthma

Asthma is a condition that affects the small tubes which carry air in and out of the lungs, an irritant usually triggers an asthma attack and irritants can vary from person to person. During an attack the muscles around the airways become increasingly narrower and the lining swells, sticky mucus can also build up in the airways which cause further narrowing and the problems associated with asthma, namely a difficulty in breathing.

There are a variety of reasons why people develop asthma, but there are certain factors that can cause it such as :

- If you have a family history of asthma or allergies
- Environmental factors such as changes in hot and cold
- Smoking during pregnancy increases the risk of your child developing asthma
- If you smoke then you are more likely to develop asthma
- Environmental pollution
- Allergies to pets
- The onset of asthma can develop after a viral infection
- Irritants found within the workplace

The most common signs and symptoms of asthma vary from person to person in severity with some people experiencing some of the symptoms all the time to some extent, while others only from time to time, they include:

- Coughing uncontrollably

- Developing a wheeze due to the restriction of the airways

- A shortness of breath

- A tight feeling around the chest

Asthma cannot be cured but it can be treated and kept under control very successfully, there are many types of medication that can help you to successfully keep your asthma under control. Medications are divided into different categories which depending on the severity of your asthma you might have to use a combination of them. Categories include

- Inhalers that prevent asthma
- Inhalers that relieve asthma
- Steroid tablets
- Spacers
- Nebulisers
- Complementary therapies

A preventer will do exactly as the name suggests help to prevent attacks of asthma, it is important to use them everyday as prescribed, even if you are feeling well. They don't help to relieve the feelings of an asthma attack such as breathlessness or tightness of the chest and most usually contain a very low dose of steroid.

Everyone who has asthma will have been prescribed a reliever; the reliever is designed to quickly ease the symptoms of asthma during an attack. The medication in the reliever will help to open the airways again making breathing much easier, it is important that if you have been prescribed an inhaler then you always make sure you have it near you.

If you have an infection and suffer from asthma then your Doctor may give you a short course of steroid treatment along with a course of antibiotics while you overcome the infection. A very few of those suffering from asthma do occasionally need to take steroids long term.

Spacers and Nebulisers are two ways that help you take your reliever medication more easily; spacers are usually given to children with asthma while Nebulisers allows you to continually inhale medication through a mask and is helpful during a particularly bad attack of asthma.

Living and coping with diabetes

Diabetes is a chronic disease that can increase the risk of developing other problems with the health. However there are many ways you can help to keep your diabetes under control and lead a relatively normal life. Living a healthy lifestyle, attending check up appointments and managing your blood sugar levels successfully, go a long way to your success in dealing with this illness.

Monitoring blood sugars

In order to maintain your diabetes successfully it is essential that you are able to monitor your own blood sugar levels. There are a variety of home machines that you are able to buy to give you accurate indications of the level. Self monitoring has the advantages of letting you be aware when your level is too low, will allow you to monitor your level during times of sickness and gives you confidence in the ability to successful keep your diabetes under control.

The best way to get accurate readings is to monitor your levels at different times during the day or week. The small machines designed to be used in the home are very easy to use and include everything you need to stay on top of the disease and help you to control it.

Get a check-up
Attending regular check ups is also a necessity, check ups are usually made every 3-months, 6-months or yearly and help to prevent complications from diabetes and make sure you are controlling it successfully during the absence of check-ups. During a check-up you will have blood tests to monitor your glucose level, test your level of cholesterol, and have your blood pressure checked and your feet and nerves. You should also schedule an eye examination to check for any damage to the back of your eyes.

Other risks
You are more at risk of developing other illnesses along with your diabetes, such as heart disease and problems with your circulation so it is imperative that you look after your overall health. Maintaining a healthy diet can go a long way to helping you keep your condition under control; you should eat at regular intervals and include low in fat while being high in fiber content. It is very important that you watch the amount of sugar you eat in your diet and also restrict the amount of salt you use in cooking and on food.

Developing an exercise routine is also good for your condition, not only will it help to keep your blood sugar level stable, but will also help you to maintain a healthy weight.

If you have diabetes then you shouldn't smoke or drink alcohol, smoking increases the risk of developing many other illnesses. If you do drink then keep it to a minimum and never drink alcohol on an empty stomach as this could lead to hypoglycemia.

You should also buy home kits for testing your level of cholesterol and blood pressure, the ideal for blood pressure is around 130/80 and your cholesterol level should be below 4.0 if you suffer from diabetes.

Preventing carpel tunnel syndrome

The bones and other tissues in your wrist help to protect your median nerve; together they form a narrow tunnel that is known as the carpel tunnel. Your median nerve is what gives you feeling in your fingers but occasionally ligaments and tendons get swollen and become painful as they press against the median nerve. When this happens your hand hurts or even becomes numb and you develop an extremely painful condition know as carpel tunnel syndrome.

Carpel tunnel syndrome most commonly affects people who do the same movements with their hands continually. Those who more at risk include typists, carpenters, grocery packers and assembly line workers, people with hobbies such as gardening, needlework, golfing and canoeing are also more at risk of developing the syndrome. It has also been linked with illnesses such as diabetes, arthritis and thyroid disease and women in the last few months of pregnancy can develop it.

The first signs that indicate you might be suffering from carpel tunnel syndrome include

- Tingling or numbness felt in your hands and fingers, especially around the index, middle fingers and thumb.
- Pain in the palm of your hand, forearm or wrist
- The pain or numbness is worse at night than it is during the day
- The pain gets worse the more you use your hands
- You have trouble gripping things and drop them more often
- Your thumb feels particularly weak

Your doctor will perform an examination of your hand, fingers and wrist to help determine whether you have carpal tunnel syndrome and may include a nerve conduction test to help the diagnosis. If carpal tunnel syndrome is diagnosed, treatment will usually consist of you having to wear a splint, and give your wrist a rest and change the way you use your wrist. The splint can help to alleviate the pain felt, particularly at night. Massaging the area of pain and putting ice onto the area can all help, as can performing stretching exercises. With treatment it is a condition that will improve, but there are some things you can do to help prevent the onset of carpel tunnel syndrome.

Increasing your awareness of how you use your hands and equipment throughout the day can make a change

Centering your work directly in front of you, your forearms should be parallel to the floor or slightly lowered

If you stand up to work then have your work bench at waist height

Make sure your hands and wrists are in line with your forearms

If you work long hours at a keyboard then titling it can help

Use proper hand and wrist movements when using a mouse and trackball

Make sure you hold your elbows in close to your sides

Never rest of the heel of your hand or wrist especially if you have them bent at an angle

Make sure that you take a slight break every 20 minutes

Do some stretching or flexing exercises every 20 minutes

Living with arthritis

While arthritis is usually considered to be a condition that affects the older generation, it can affect people of any age. It can affect any part of the body and there are thought to be over 200 different forms of the disease. However, the three most common types of arthritis are osteoarthritis, rheumatoid and juvenile arthritis.

People who are affected by arthritis can go through many different feelings ranging from anger, frustration, worries for the future and concern about dependency. For the younger person affected by the disease feelings such as how other people will see you is a main concern, while the disease can be debilitating and so not easy to be positive about the outlook, people do come to terms with the condition. In order to come to terms with the disease you can

Talk about your feelings and fears – getting your feelings out in the open is essential to coping with your illness. Talking can relive the feelings of anxiety and stress you feel about your condition and how others see you. Your confidant can be your doctor, a friend or family member or someone that is suffering from arthritis themselves.

Learn how to relax and de-stress – many people who suffer from arthritis get stressed easily and are unable to relax. You should learn routines that allow you to relax quickly and easily or find an activity or hobby that you could take part in to ease and forget your stress.

Seek help from a professional – if you don't feel you can talk to a family member or friend then seek help from a professional. This could be a counselor, doctor, social worker or your local citizen's advice.

One of the most debilitating aspects of arthritis is the persistent pain it brings to the sufferer. However sufferers do seem to manage to keep the pain under control to a level where it doesn't interfere too much with their day-to-day living. Here are some ways to help you deal with and manage the pain associated with arthritis.

Keep a note of the best time to take medication in order to get the best benefit

Notice when cold, heat and getting rest helps the most

See which form of exercise works best for you and when to do them

Keep practicing relaxation techniques

Take a pain management course

Purchase a device such as the TENS unit to help manage your pain

Consider hypnosis or acupuncture treatment

Attend pain clinics recommended by you Doctor.

These are just some of the ways that people have been known to successfully manage their arthritis and of course you should discuss ways to help you with your doctor. You doctor will also be able to advise you of clinics in your area that you can attend to learn how to deal more effectively with the disease and the pain that it brings.

Are you at risk from Alzheimer's?

There is no one single cause of Alzheimer's disease, Alzheimer's is brought on by varying factors with each person affected being different. However, the biggest two factors which increase the risk of you developing Alzheimer's are the advancement of age and heredity. Your degree of mental fitness and your environment are also thought to play a part to some extent - although this and several other theories have not yet been proven..

Who gets Alzheimer's?
By the time you reach the age of 65, roughly 5 in 100 people have developed the disease, by the age of 80 the odds have jumped to 1 in 5 and almost half of all people at the age of 90 have some signs of dementia. Alzheimer's isn't strictly limited to those over the age of 65; much younger people have been affected by it. It is a disease that is thought to occur in women more than men, but the main reason for this is simply that women tend to live longer than men.

Alzheimer's and heredity
There has proven to be a heredity link to Alzheimer's in roughly 3% of all cases of the disease. Heredity is thought to occur when the onset of the disease has occurred at an early age, with about 40% of people who developed the disease before the age of 65 having family members affected by the disease. This does not mean that having a family member with Alzheimer's will guarantee being affected by it. Quite the contrary, although those with affected family members are at a slightly higher risk than others, there are still measures that can be taken to help avoid the onset of Alzheimer's.

Avoiding Alzheimer's
Many believe that the environment in which you live can make a difference as to whether you are more susceptible to developing Alzheimer's. Research is currently being conducted as to whether exposure to certain metals is a contributing factor to developing the disease. Many experts have tied aluminum as a possible cause of the disease and suggest that antiperspirant deodorants are avoided due to their high aluminum content.

Many doctors also believe that one's state of mental health plays a large part in the onset of the disease. The sharper one keeps oneself, the less susceptible one is to the disease. However, there is not currently any evidence to suggest that staying mentally fit will make a difference one way or the other.

There are thought to be many other factors that could lead to the onset of Alzheimer's, but additional research is needed due to there being a lot of conflicting evidence. Factors to consider include, head trauma, various viral infections, a history of downs syndrome in the family, smoking and thyroid disease.

The future of Alzheimer's
Unfortunately, there is not currently any particular test that doctors can use to indicate who may be more susceptible of developing the disease. The primary goal in research right now is to understand better the mechanisms of the disease with the hope of one day being able to predict those people who are more susceptible to Alzheimer's before the disease actually sets in. By doing so, scientists and doctors believe that it could lead to developments of treatment to delay the onset of Alzheimer's.

Dealing with allergies

It is possible to develop an allergy to almost anything; this could be a smell, food, medication or reactions to dander found on animals. An allergy can range from nothing more than an annoying itch to the more serious of going into shock after developing a severe reaction. Allergies are usually divided into different categories that include:

Eczema and urticaria – these are allergies which affect the skin; they include allergic skin rashes such as nettle rash and hives.

Hay fever – this condition causes reactions such as runny nose, sneezing, coughing and sore eyes during the summer months.

Venom allergies – these are reactions to stinging insects and snakes.

Adverse food reactions – people can be allergic to many different types of food.

Allergy to drugs – certain medications can cause a reaction in people; the usual reactions to drugs include a rash, sickness and stomach problems.

Anaphylaxis – a severe and sudden intense allergic reaction that affects the whole body.

Asthma – an allergic reaction that commonly affects the breathing.

Eye allergies – this can vary from very mild irritation to severe conjunctivitis.

Diagnosing allergies

If your doctor believes that you may have an allergy then steps will need to be taken to identify what is causing it, the allergen. The most common way of finding the allergen is to perform a skin prick test. The skin prick test is quick and relatively painless and the results are known immediately.

A small needle is used to gently prick your skin with the allergen; the test will usually be conducted on your forearm. You are determined to be allergic to the allergen if your skin becomes red, sore and itchy around the area the needle was inserted. It is also usual for the area to come up in a welt. If you have had no reaction to the allergen after a period of roughly 20 minutes then you aren't allergic to that allergen.

If it is suspected that you have dermatitis - a form of eczema then you will normally be given a skin patch test, this test relies on taping patches with various allergens underneath aluminum discs. The discs are usually kept in place for a period of 48 hours and then assessed by a dermatologist for allergic changes.

Severe cases

In severe cases of allergy you might be required to have a challenge test to be performed in hospital. The suspected allergens are then introduced directly into the lungs or nose and the allergic reaction is then measured. If it is suspected that you might be allergic to food or foods then a double blind placebo test may be used. The food or foods that are thought to cause a reaction are given in a capsule under supervision, and then you wait to see if you develop a reaction to it. This type of test however is only done in extreme circumstances because despite it being the most reliable way it is also the most time consuming.

Alter Your Acne Problems

One of those dreaded 4-letter words is acne because it often calls to mind dreaded terms like: zits, pimples, whiteheads, blackheads, blemishes, clogged pores and unsightly skin. However, dreaded doesn't have to mean hopeless, because there is hope.

Main causes of acne are known and often easily treatable. For example, blemishes often appear because of body chemistry changes during teen years, menstrual cycles and menopause. Other reasons are frequently due to too much bacteria clogging pores and over scrubbing of face to rid it of acne.

Treatments include over the counter anti-acne over-the-counter solutions, prescription drugs and natural remedies. Some popular actions to take right away at home are:

1. Get an exfoliating cleanser and some anti-acne soap from the local drugstore or supermarket and wash your face gently with them every

day. For best results, wash as soon as you get up in the morning and right before you go to bed at night. And do not squeeze pimples.

2. Get an anti-acne facial mask at the drugstore or find a honey facial mask, for the disinfecting and healing qualities. Use the mask up to two times a week.

3. Check with your healthcare provider about adding a multivitamin to your daily routine and a chromium supplement.

4. Keep hair back and away from your face, especially your forehead.

5. Drink plenty of liquids daily; eight glasses of water is recommended most. And eat foods rich in beta-carotene and vitamin A to help with skin repair like carrots.

6. Avoid putting makeup, paints, etc. on your face, unless they are water soluble or marked as noncomedogenic types – and even then, go very light. And use a fresh, clean pillow case every day.

7. If you go out in the sun, apply a minimal sunscreen with SPF 15. And when possible, choose one that's a noncomedogenic or nonacnegenic type so it doesn't clog pores. Add a hat and sunglasses. And skip tanning beds.

Also in order to clear acne, it helps to clear up acne rumors. Here are some popular issues to clear up:

- Greasy foods, stress and chocolates can cause and increase acne problems. This is a myth. There is no scientific connection here between these elements.

- Squeezing your pimples can help get rid of them. This is also untrue. Squeezing can actually make matters worse, forcing infection further below the skin's surface and can even cause scarring.

- Being out in the sun can help dry up acne. This is not true. Too much sun can actually make things worse, adding dryness and irritation to your skin, not to mention wrinkles and skin cancer later in life.

Lowering your blood pressure

You should have your blood pressure tested at least every 2 years, because high blood pressure can lead to problems such as damaging your blood vessels. High blood pressure can increase your risk of heart disease, heart attack, developing kidney failure and stroke. Having your blood pressure checked takes only a few minutes and should there be a problem your doctor can treat it and recommend changes to your lifestyle that you should follow. Here are some simple tips to making changes in your lifestyle to keep your blood pressure within a normal range.

Stop smoking
If you smoke then you should try to quit, when you inhale the smoke from cigarettes and other tobacco products, your blood vessels become restricted and you will have a faster heartbeat. If your heart beats faster than this causes a temporary rise in your blood pressure, by quitting smoking you not only help to lower your blood pressure but you also reduce the risk of heart disease and heart attack.

Lose weight
Losing weight and getting enough exercise can help towards keeping your blood pressure down. If you are carrying too much weight around your heart will have to work harder and faster and this can cause your blood pressure to rise which increases your chances of developing heart disease and stroke.

Limit your alcohol intake
Limiting the amount of alcohol you drink is also important, in some people alcohol raises their blood pressure by a lot, while others it doesn't seem to affect as much. You should drink no more than 1 glass of wine per day or one can of beer and if your blood pressure does rise through drinking, then you should quit drinking altogether.

Avoid excessive sodium
Some people can be affected by sodium and it causes their blood pressure to rise. If you have been diagnosed with high blood pressure then it is important to reduce the amount of sodium in your diet. You shouldn't add extra salt to your food and always check food labels for the amount of sodium foods contain.

Lower stress levels
If you live a very stressful life and easily become stressed then this can cause your blood pressure to rise, it is important to learn ways of dealing with stress and not let it build up. There are many self-help techniques that you can learn to help you combat stress, such as meditation, deep breathing exercises, yoga and visualization.

Blood pressure medication
If your doctor has diagnosed you as having high blood pressure then along with making changes to your lifestyle - the most effective way of dealing with it - they might also prescribe medication. There are many different types of medication used in the treatment of high blood pressure. In some cases, if your condition can only be controlled by medication, then it could mean that you have to take medication for the rest of your life to help keep your blood pressure under control. However the earlier you start making changes to your lifestyle towards leading a healthier life, through stopping smoking, getting enough exercise and eating healthy, the better your chances that you won't need to be on medication for life.

Chapter IV: Natural Healing Powers

Alternative Medicine Basics

Alternative medicine is a term that refers to medical practices outside of conventional medicine. Alternative solutions are sometimes new and untested in the scientific realm of conventional medicine, stamped with approval of the federal government. Also, they sometimes focus around or contain a religious, spiritual or metaphysical element. Here are some popular alternative medicinal solutions.

Acupuncture – This is the art of inserting tiny needles underneath the skin that stimulate targeted body spots. Acupuncture is most often used to relieve pain and heal the body.

Apitherapy – Better known as Bee Therapy, this practice makes use of honey and venom from the honeybee for treatments. Popular ones for health and beauty products and healing treatments are raw honey, bee pollen, royal jelly and propolis.

Biofeedback – This refers to a machine that gives feedback on the body. The feedback helps healthcare providers chart bodily functions to help with treatment. These machines are used to chart internal functions with more accuracy than a human alone is capable of, and the results are used to determine and then gauge how well the treatment is working. Biofeedback has been used to help people with their emotional disorders, digestive disorders, stress, migraines and heart irregularities. The machine alerts people to the idea of how their own emotions and thoughts can come into play with regards to illness and treatment options.

Chiropractics – This form of back treatment has been around for awhile and focuses on the vertebrae not being aligned properly, thus contributing to a variety of pain, illnesses and diseases. Many also focus on stress, overall health and lifestyle. In general, a chiropractor applies pressure in small amounts to various vertebrae, helping them realign. Plus many help treat common diseases like asthma, troubled backs and arthritis.

Feng Shui - This is a philosophy that is said to bring harmony into lives, that features not only the four basic elements of earth, fire, water and air, but a fifth; metal. By aligning these elements throughout clutter-free homes, work, outdoor and other environments, peace and tranquility are said to follow.

Healing Crystals – These minerals turned crystalline are said to boast certain healing powers. For example, ancient grave sites house them as a means of protection in the afterlife. In the modern world, many believe these crystals house healing power. For example, to treat stomach pain, some healers place charged quartz on the lower abdomen area to help restore energy there.

Herbal Remedies – Applying herbs, either home grown or store bought, to certain ailments helps with healing for many conditions. Among popular treatments are a half-and-half solution of witch hazel and water to help clear up acne, lavender scented oils and candles to sooth stress and garlic on top of warts to remove them.

There are many more alternative medicine treatments out there. Search your favorite search engine for more.

The Benefits of Chinese Medicine

Chinese medicine is a whole holistic system that can lead to a healthier, happier and more stress free way of living. It is a system that people have benefited from for over twenty-three centuries and is used to diagnose, treat and prevent a wide variety or illnesses and problems.

The different aspects that make up Chinese medicine all basically rely on the same principle, Yin and Yang. This is basically opposites attract, such as night and day, cold and warm, inner and outer. The basis behind it is to restore harmony and peace to the mind and body; the Chinese believe that by doing so we can eliminate many diseases and illnesses.

Qi is the life force that flows uninterrupted throughout the body, similar to blood throwing throughout the veins. It is when there is a disruption in this Qi that problems and illness occurs; restoring the flow of the Qi restores harmony and dissolves the symptoms of illness.

The two main components of Chinese medicine are acupuncture and herbal remedies.

Acupuncture

Acupuncture focuses on the Qi that flows throughout the body; it flows through points known as meridian points. While it is flowing freely we are healthy and happy, but if the channels should become blocked then the Qi stagnates and this leads to symptoms of various illnesses depending on where the Qi is blocked. It works by the acupuncturist restoring the normal flow of the Qi by stimulating certain points on the body.

Herbal medicine

Chinese herbal medicine is usually dispensed after acupuncture treatment although it can be used as a standalone. There are over a thousand common herbs that are used in combinations for various problems and illnesses. There are two main types of herbal remedies that are commonly used, these are "food herbs" and are generally eaten as part of the diet and are mainly used for prevention of disease and illness and maintenance. "Medicinal herbs" are usually prescribed by a Doctor of Chinese medicine and are specially prepared for the patient based on the individuals needs. The formula is made up from the patient's medical condition, the environment and the constitution of the person. Medicinal herbs are usually given alongside acupuncture treatment and used in conjunction with the "re-balancing" effects of acupuncture treatment.

The benefits of Chinese medicine are numerous and is has been thought to have helped many physical conditions along with affective disorders and increases mental clarity, here are just a few of the conditions it has been known to successfully treat.

- Sinusitis, bronchitis and asthma
- Conjunctivitis and cataracts
- Stroke, sciatica and osteoarthritis
- Faster recovery from injury
- Improved circulation
- Relief from stress and anxiety
- Relief from pain
- Strengthening of the immune system
- Addictions, phobias and eating disorders

Improve Your Health with Aromatherapy

Aromatherapy, a term created in 1920, involves the use of essential oils that are compounds in their purist state. The oils are concentrated liquids derived from plants through a variety of means: distillation, solvent extraction or expression processing. And the resulting oils are then used as treatment for a variety of ailments and healing.

Aromatherapy was actually coined because of Mr. Rene Maurice Gattefosse. While he was conducting research about how oils might aid healing, his arm caught fire and subsequently poured lavender oil onto it by accidental, which in turn caused the arm to heal faster, leaving no scar.   Since that time, many have delved into how aromatherapy can help with physical and emotional healing.

Popular Uses

Some common uses for aromatherapy oils are as scents for homes and offices to help trigger relaxing feelings from occupants and to also help get rid of unwanted smells and germs. For example, lighting candles and burning wax chips made with aromatherapy oils can help rid a kitchen of smelly fried onion and other food smells.

A light fragrance can help welcome people home after a long day at the office. Popular scents are bergamot, eucalyptus, lavender, jasmine and rose.

Some of the oils can help fight bacteria, like lavender oil. And others, like camphor and menthol can help increase your metabolism and endocrine system, improve your central nervous system and boost your immune system to fight colds.

Other aromatherapy oils are used for massage treatments, too. Absorbed by the skin and muscles, the oils activate thermal receptors that result in warm relaxing feelings and calmness in the muscle groups.

And still other aromatherapy oils are used as topical aids to aid in the destruction of microbes and other fungi; the oils are simply applied to the skin. And other oils are taken internally where they can help improve antiseptic activity, stimulate your immune system and work as a diuretic aid.

Safety Precautions

When deciding about the uses of aromatherapy for your ailments and healing, use the following guidelines as precautionary measures:

- Pure essential aromatherapy oils can be very strong and harmful to animals, children and you. So check labels carefully before using aromatherapy products, and consult your healthcare provider if needed. And do not use in pure oils undiluted on your skin.

- Do not use aromatherapy oils if you are pregnant, or have epilepsy or asthma.

- Test the ingredients and sample a drop or two first to check for allergic reactions.

- Only use aromatherapy oils in small amounts as they can cause burning of the eyes and other negative reactions.

How to Cure Depression without Drugs

On the face of it, this question of trying to cure depression without drugs seems to be futile, especially these days when most people have gotten used to the idea of being treated with prescriptions drugs. But many people are successfully turning away from prescription drugs and finding alternative methods of treatment – without drugs. Those suffering from depression, too, are taking recourse to drugless therapies, which generally do not cause any side-effects and are typically much more economical.

Low light blues

Depending upon the cause of your depression, you will need to choose an appropriate type of therapy. If your depressive disorder manifests itself in winter, when days are short and daylight is sparse, you may effectively make use of phototherapy. Bright light therapy, or blue light therapy, given with the help of a light box, is believed to reduce or remove the cause of this type of depression.

Psychotherapy

Psychotherapy will be helpful in cases in which psychological factors like skewed thought patterns are identified to have caused depression. In such cases, psychotherapy or counseling will work better if there is good understanding and a solid rapport between the counselor and the patient. Depending on the severity of the disorder, long and frequent counseling sessions may be necessary due to the patient's distorted thought patterns. Thought patterns, personal relationships, and low self-esteem must be corrected. Self-loathing has to be converted onto self-love and stress has to be lowered or eliminated and so on. By and large, the most important thing is the approach the counselor brings to the table as well as the counselor-patient relationship.

Exercise

Physical exercise is also considered to be very good as a cure for depression, particularly when it is combined with psychotherapy. It is an effective method to get rid of excessive stress, which may cause depression. Although it may be rather difficult to make severely depressed people physically active, persistent efforts aimed at motivating them to get involved in regular physical activities are likely to be successful. In practice, group physical activities are known to alleviate depression by cutting at its root causes like traumatic breakdown in personal relationships and stress-related factors.

Food and Diet

In certain cases of depression, dietary supplements like those which are rich in Omega-3 fatty acids (particularly those found naturally in oily fish) work as a cure. Products containing chocolate and Vitamin B-12 are proven to work as antidepressants. Some herbal substances are also found to be effective. When depression occurs due to misuse of alcohol and other intoxicants, caffeine, sleep-inducing drugs and sedatives, the obvious cure lies in teaching the patient not to use these depression triggers.

Meditation and prayer

Meditation and deep breathing exercises are being increasingly used as a means of treating depression without drugs. These have produced results proven to be very effective especially when practiced regularly over a considerable period of time. The calming effect of meditation on the mind has a positive impact for depression sufferers. Prayer and spirituality may also be useful in this regard.

Rehabilitation of depressed people is a family and social responsibility. Often times a depressed person is just looking for the attention of loved ones. Attempts to treat depression by drugs alone will not be successful. For this reason, the stigma that is associated with mental illnesses like depression has to be discarded. Loved ones must not discriminate against depressed people because this can make the problem worse. Love an support is the best way to start looking for a cure for depression.

Sleeping your way to health

Most of us don't realize the true value that sleep can have on our bodies and minds and the majority of us don't get enough of it. While for some of us this is due to suffering from a sleep disorder such as insomnia, others just stay up too late and have commitments which require us to get up early. Getting enough quality sleep is essential to getting us through our day but also for our overall health.

One of the biggest things that lack of sleep has on our bodies is our hormones; various hormones in our body work together and have an effect on our health. When we suffer from lack of sleep we begin to crave more carbohydrates and sugar, our blood sugar levels will also fluctuate. If we don't get enough sleep it can cause problems with out adrenal glands, the adrenal glands regulate your body's health, when our adrenal glands start suffering, and we start to suffer.

One of the main problems being an increase in hormone cortisol, cortisol helps us to resist stress, maintain our blood pressure and our moods are dependant on it. However if there is an increase in cortisol then it can cause adverse reactions within our body and is not good for us.

So what can we do to ensure that we get enough sleep? Here are some tips to help

- Avoid eating before going to bed – if possible do not eat after 7pm, the later you eat the less time your body has to digest food before you go to bed. Instead of resting your body will spend all night digesting the food you ate. Also going to bed on a full stomach will lead to you feeling uncomfortable and tossing and turning all night long.
- Get enough exercise throughout the day – if you aren't getting enough exercise throughout the day then you aren't going to be tired. Getting regular exercise not only gets you fitter but also helps you to get a good nights rest.
- Dim your lights – just as the sun streaming through your window first thing in the morning starts your day off by energizing you, dimming your lights at night can encourage your body to slow down and unwind.
- Buy a suitable mattress – if you are having trouble getting comfortable at night in bed then consider buying a new mattress, if your mattress is

old and worn this could be the reason you are tossing and turning all night.

- Have a schedule and keep to it – develop a healthy internal clock by getting yourself into a routine. Get up at the same time every morning and go to bed at the same time.
- Avoid taking naps – where possible stay awake and don't take a nap during the day, taking a nap during the day confuses your internal clock and you are not as tired when it comes to going to bed.
- Keep your bedroom relaxed – avoid turning your bedroom into an office, don't put a desk or computer in there and be tempted to work. If you have work in there you are more than likely going to thinking of the things you have done or should have done and this can keep you awake.
- A hot drink – try winding down with a hot drink before going to bed, of course give this time to go through your body before lying down for the night, otherwise you will awaken with the need to go to the bathroom. Preferably make cocoa with hot milk but avoid coffee and tea.